Air Fryer Menu

50 Super Easy And Stress-Free Recipes For Your Air Fryer

Elena Simmons

Table of Content

Introduction

There are many kinds of foods that you can cook using an air fryer, but there are also certain types that are not suited for it. Avoid cooking ingredients, which can be steamed, like beans and carrots. You also cannot fry foods covered in heavy batter in this appliance.

Aside from the above mentioned, you can cook most kinds of ingredients using an air fryer. You can use it to cook foods covered in light flour or breadcrumbs. You can cook a variety of vegetables in the appliance, such as cauliflower, asparagus, zucchini, kale, peppers, and corn on the cob. You can also use it to cook frozen foods and home prepared meals by following a different set of instructions for these purposes.

An air fryer also comes with another useful feature - the separator. It allows you to cook multiple dishes at a time. Use the separator to divide ingredients in the pan or basket. You have to make sure that all ingredients have the same temperature setting so that everything will cook evenly at the same time.

The Benefits of Air fryer

It is important to note that air fried foods are still fried. Unless you've decided to eliminate the use of oils in cooking, you must still be cautious about the food you eat. Despite that, it clearly presents a better and healthier option than deep-frying. It helps you avoid unnecessary fats and oils, which makes it an ideal companion when you intend to lose weight. It offers a lot more benefits, which include the following:

•   It is convenient and easy to use, plus, it's easy to clean.

•   It doesn't give off unwanted smells when cooking.

•   You can use it to prepare a variety of meals.

- It can withstand heavy cooking.

- It is durable and made of metal and high-grade plastic.

- Cooking using this appliance is not as messy as frying in a traditional way. You don't have to worry

about greasy spills and stains in the kitchen.

Breakfast

17.   Spaghetti Squash Casserole Cups

Preparation time: 10 minutes

Cooking time: 15 minutes Servings: 2

INGREDIENTS

- 12 oz spaghetti squash
- 1 carrot, grated
- 1 egg
- 1/3 teaspoon chili flakes
- 1 onion, chopped

DIRECTIONS

1.   Peel the spaghetti squash and grate it.

2.   Mix up together the spaghetti squash and carrot.

3.   Beat the egg and stir it carefully.

4.   After this, add the chili flakes and chopped onion.

5.   Stir it.

6.   Place the mixture in the air fryer basket and cook the casserole for 15 minutes at 365 F.

7.   When the casserole is cooked – chill it till the room temperature.

8.   Serve it!

NUTRITION: Calories 119, Fat 3.2, Fiber 1.9,

Carbs 20.1, Protein 4.7

18.   Chopped Kale with Ground Beef

Preparation time: 12 minutes Cooking time: 16 minutes Servings: 4

INGREDIENTS

- 12 oz kale
- 1 cup ground beef
- ½ teaspoon salt
- ½ onion, diced
- 1 teaspoon ground paprika
- ¼ teaspoon minced garlic
- 1 teaspoon dried dill
- 1 teaspoon olive oil
- 1 oz almonds, crushed

DIRECTIONS

1.   Mix up together the salt, diced onion, ground paprika, minced garlic, and dried dill in the mixing bowl.

2.   Add the olive oil and stir carefully.

3.   After this, place the ground beef in the air fryer basket.

4.   Add the olive oil mixture. Stir it carefully.

5.   Cook the ground beef for 13 minutes at 370 F. Stir it time to time.

6.   Meanwhile, chop the kale.

7.   Add the kale and crushed almonds in the ground beef.

8.   Stir it and cook for 3 minutes more at 350 F.

9.   Then transfer the cooked meal in the serving bowls and serve!

NUTRITION: Calories 180, Fat 7.5, Fiber 2.7,

Carbs 12.2, Protein 17.2

19.   Bacon Wrapped Chicken Fillet

Preparation time: 15 minutes Cooking time: 15 minutes Servings: 6

INGREDIENTS

- 15 oz chicken fillet
- 6 oz bacon, sliced
- ½ teaspoon salt
- 1 teaspoon paprika
- 1 tablespoon olive oil
- 1 garlic clove, chopped

DIRECTIONS

1.   Rub the chicken fillet with the salt, paprika, garlic clove and olive oil.

2.   Wrap the rubbed chicken fillet in the bacon and secure gently with the toothpicks.

3.   Place the chicken fillets in the air fryer basket.

4.   Cook the chicken for 15 minutes at

380 F. Stir the chicken every 5 minutes.

5.   Then slice the cooked chicken fillet and serve!

NUTRITION: Calories 310, Fat 19.5, Fiber 0.1,

Carbs 0.8, Protein 31.1

21.   Eggs in Avocado Preparation time: 10 minutes
Cooking time: 7 minutes Servings: 2

INGREDIENTS

- 1 avocado, pitted
- 2 eggs
- ½ ground black pepper
- ¾ teaspoon salt

DIRECTIONS

1.   Cut the avocado into the halves.

2.   Then sprinkle the avocado with the black
pepper and salt.

3.   Beat the eggs and place them in the

avocado halve's wholes.

4. Place the avocado in the air fryer basket.

5. Cook the meal for 7 minutes at 380 F.

6. When the eggs are cooked – the meal is ready to eat.

7. Serve it immediately!

NUTRITION: Calories 268, Fat 24, Fiber 6.7,

Carbs 9, Protein 7.5

24. Turkey Tortillas

Preparation time: 5 minutes

Cooking time: 14 minutes Servings: 4

INGREDIENTS

• 1 pound turkey breast, skinless, boneless, ground and browned

• 4 corn tortillas

• Cooking spray

• 1 cup cherry tomatoes, halved

• 1 cup kalamata olives, pitted and halved

• 1 cup corn

• 1 cup baby spinach

- 1 cup cheddar cheese, shredded
- Salt and black pepper to the taste

DIRECTIONS

1.   Divide the meat, tomatoes and the other ingredients except the cooking spray on each tortilla, roll and grease them with the cooking spray

2.   Preheat the air fryer at 350 degrees F, put the tortillas in the air fryer's basket, cook for 7 minutes on each side, divide between plates and serve for breakfast.

NUTRITION: Calories 244, Fat 11, Fiber 4, Carbs 5, Protein 7

25.   Turkey and Peppers Bowls Preparation time: 5 minutes Cooking time: 20 minutes

Servings: 4

INGREDIENTS

- 1 red bell pepper, cut into strips
- 1-pound turkey breast, skinless, boneless, ground
- 4 eggs, whisked

- Salt and black pepper to the taste

- 1 cup corn

- 1 cup black olives, pitted and halved

- 1 cup mild salsa

- Cooking spray

DIRECTIONS

1. Heat up the air fryer at 350 degrees F, grease it with cooking spray, add the meat, peppers and the other ingredients, toss and cook for 20 minutes.

2. Divide into bowls and serve for breakfast.

NUTRITION: Calories 229, Fat 13, Fiber 3, Carbs 4, Protein 7

26. Potato Casserole Preparation time: 5 minutes Cooking time: 20 minutes Servings: 4

INGREDIENTS

- 1 pound gold potatoes, peeled and cubed

- 4 eggs, whisked

- 1 teaspoon chili powder

- 1 cup carrots, peeled and sliced

- 1 cup black olives, pitted and halved

- 1 cup mozzarella, shredded

- 2 tablespoons butter, melted

- A pinch of salt and black pepper

DIRECTIONS

1.   Heat up your air fryer at 320 degrees F, grease with the butter, and combine the potatoes with the eggs, chili and the other ingredients except the mozzarella and toss.

2.   Sprinkle the mozzarella on top, cook for

20 minutes, divide between plates and serve for breakfast.

NUTRITION: Calories 240, Fat 9, Fiber 2, Carbs 4, Protein 8

27. Chives Quinoa Bowls Preparation time: 5 minutes Cooking time: 20 minutes Servings: 4

INGREDIENTS

- 1 tablespoon olive oil
- 1 cup quinoa
- 2 cups almond milk
- 2 tablespoons chives, chopped
- ½ cup kalamata olives, pitted and halved
- ½ cup mozzarella, shredded
- ½ teaspoon turmeric powder
- Salt and black pepper to the taste

DIRECTIONS

1.   Heat up the air fryer with the oil at 350 degrees F, combine the quinoa with the milk, chives and the other ingredients inside, cook for 20 minutes, divide into bowls and serve for breakfast.

NUTRITION: Calories 221, Fat 8, Fiber 3, Carbs 4, Protein 8

28. Creamy Almond Rice Preparation time: 10 minutes Cooking time: 20 minutes Servings: 4

INGREDIENTS

- 2 cups almond milk
- 1 cup white rice
- ½ cup almonds, chopped
- ½ teaspoon vanilla extract
- ½ teaspoon almond extract
- ½ cup heavy cream
- Cooking spray

DIRECTIONS

1. Heat up your air fryer with the oil at 350 degrees F, grease it with the cooking spray, add the rice, milk and the other ingredients inside, toss, cook everything for 20 minutes, divide into bowls and serve.

NUTRITION: Calories 231, Fat 11, Fiber 3, Carbs 5, Protein 8

15.   Kale Quiche with Eggs

Preparation time: 10 minutes Cooking time: 18 minutes Servings: 6

INGREDIENTS

- 1 cup kale
- 3 eggs
- 2 oz bacon, chopped, cooked
- 1 sweet potato, grated
- ½ teaspoon thyme
- ½ teaspoon ground black pepper
- ½ teaspoon ground paprika
- ½ cup coconut milk
- 1 onion, chopped
- 1 teaspoon olive oil

DIRECTIONS

1.   Chop the kale roughly and place it in the blender.

2.   Blend it gently.

3.   Then transfer the blended kale in the mixing bowl.

4.   Add the grated potato and thyme.

5.   Sprinkle the mixture with the ground black pepper and ground paprika.

6.   Add coconut   milk and chopped onion.

7.   Pour the olive oil into the air fryer basket.

8.   Then place the kale mixture in the air fryer basket,

9.   Beat the eggs in the separate bowl and whisk well.

10.   Pour the whisked eggs over the kale mixture. Add bacon.

11.   Cook the quiche for 18 minutes at 350 F.

12.   When the time is over – chill the quiche little and serve!

NUTRITION: Calories 166, Fat 11.8, Fiber 1.8,

Carbs 8.5, Protein 7.7

16. Breakfast Bacon Hash

Preparation time: 10 minutes Cooking time: 19 minutes Servings: 2

INGREDIENTS

- 1 oz bacon, chopped
- 1 carrot
- 1 apple
- 1 teaspoon olive oil
- ½ teaspoon salt
- ¼ teaspoon thyme

DIRECTIONS

1. Put the chopped bacon in the air fryer basket.

2. Add salt and stir it gently.

3. Cook the bacon for 4 minutes at 365 F.

4. Peel the carrot and grate it.

5. Add the grated carrot.

6. Then grate the apple and add the carrot mixture too.

7. Stir it carefully.

8. Sprinkle the bacon hash with the thyme and stir gently again.

9. Cook the bacon hash for 15 minutes at 365 F.

10. Stir it carefully and serve!

NUTRITION: Calories 168, Fat 8.5, Fiber 3.5, Carbs 18.7, Protein 5.8

Mains, Sides Recipes

137. Medium-Rare Beef Steak

Cooking Time: 6 minutes Servings: 1 INGREDIENTS

- 1-3cm thick beef steak

- 1tablespoon olive oil

- Salt and pepper to taste

DIRECTIONS

1.   Preheat your air fryer to 350°Fahrenheit. Coat the steak with olive oil on both sides and season both sides with salt and pepper. Place the steak into the baking tray of air fryer and cook for 3- minutes per side.

NUTRITION: Calories: 445, Total Fat: 21g, Carbs: 0g, Protein: 59.6g

138. Spicy Duck Legs Cooking Time: 30 minutes Servings: 2

INGREDIENTS

- 2duck legs, bone-in, skin on

- Salt and pepper to taste

- 1teaspoon five spice powder

- 1tablespoon herbs that you like such as thyme, parsley, etc., chopped

DIRECTIONS

1.   Rub the spices over duck legs. Place duck legs in the air fryer and cook for 25- minutes at 325°Fahrenheit. Then air fries them at 400°Fahrenheit for 5-minutes.

NUTRITION: Calories: 207,   Total   Fat: 10.6g, Carbs: 1.9g, Protein: 25g

139. Stuffed Turkey Cooking Time: 63 minutes Servings: 6

INGREDIENTS

- 1whole turkey, bone-in, with skin
- 2celery stalks, chopped
- 1lemon, sliced
- Fresh oregano leaves, chopped
- 1cup fresh parsley, minced
- 1teaspoon sage leaves, dry
- 2cups turkey broth
- 4cloves garlic, minced
- 1onion, chopped
- 2eggs

- 1½ lbs sage sausage

- 4tablespoons butter

DIRECTIONS

1.   Preheat your air fryer to 390°Fahrenheit. In a pan over medium- heat melt 2 ½ tablespoons of butter. Add the sausage (remove sausage meat from skinand mash. Cook sausage meat in the pan for 8- minutes and stir. Add in celery, onions, garlic, and sage and cook for an additional 10-minutes, stir to combine. Remove sausage mixture from heat and add the broth. In a bowl, whisk eggs and two tablespoons   of parsley. Pour egg mixture into sausage mix and stir. This will be the stuffing for your turkey. Fill the turkey with the stuffing mix. In a separate bowl, combine the remaining butter with parsley, oregano, salt, and pepper and rub this mix onto turkey skin. Place the turkey inside the air fryer and cook for 45- minutes. Garnish with lemon slices.

NUTRITION: Calories: 1046, Total Fat: 69.7g, Carbs: 12.7g, Protein: 91.5g

140. Turkey Breast with Maple Mustard Glaze

Cooking Time: 42 minutes Servings: 6

INGREDIENTS

- 5lbs. of boneless turkey breast
- ¼ Maple Syrup sugar-free
- 2tablespoons Dijon Mustard
- 1tablespoon butter
- 2olive oil
- Dried herbs: sage, thyme, smoked paprika
- Salt and pepper to taste

DIRECTIONS

1.   Preheat air fryer to 350°Fahrenheit. Rub turkey breasts with olive oil. Combine the spices and season the turkey on the

outside with this mix of spices. Place the turkey in air fryer and cook for 25- minutes. Turn over and cook for an additional 12-minutes more. In a small saucepan over medium heat mix the maple syrup, mustard, and butter. Brush the turkey with the glaze in an upright position. Air fry for 5-minutes or until turkey breasts is golden in color.

NUTRITION: Calories: 464, Total Fat: 10g, Carbs: 25g, Protein: 64.6g

141. Garlic Chicken Kebab Cooking Time: 10 minutes Servings: 2

INGREDIENTS

- 1lb. chicken fillet, cut into small pieces
- 1tablespoon garlic, minced
- ½ cup plain yogurt
- 1tablespoon olive oil
- Juice of one lime
- 1teaspoon turmeric powder
- 1teaspoon red chili powder
- 1teaspoon black pepper
- 1tablespoon chicken masala

DIRECTIONS

1.   Mix the yogurt and spices in a bowl. Add the oil and squeeze half a lime into it and stir. Coat the

chicken pieces with mixture one at a time. Marinate the chicken pieces in the fridge for 2 hours. Preheat your air fryer to 356°Fahrenheit. Place the grill pan into the air fryer and put the chicken pieces into it. Cook chicken for 10-minutes.

NUTRITION: Calories: 355, Total Fat: 12.7g, Carbs: 7.8g, Protein: 49.6g

130. Mustard Pork Balls

Servings: 4

INGREDIENTS

- 7-ounces of minced pork

- 1teaspoon of organic honey

- 1teaspoon Dijon mustard

- 1tablespoon cheddar cheese, grated

- 1/3 cup onion, diced

- Salt and pepper to taste

- A handful of fresh basil, chopped

- 1teaspoon garlic puree

DIRECTIONS

1. In a bowl, mix the meat with all of the seasonings and form balls.

2.   Place the pork balls into air fryer and cook for 15-minutes at 392°Fahrenheit.

NUTRITION: Calories: 121, Total Fat: 6.8g, Carbs: 2.7g, Protein: 11.3g

131. Garlic Pork Chops Cooking Time: 16 minutes Servings: 4

INGREDIENTS

- 4pork chops
- 1tablespoon coconut butter
- 2teaspoons minced garlic cloves
- 1tablespoon coconut butter
- 2teaspoons parsley, chopped
- salt and pepper to taste

DIRECTIONS

1.   Preheat your air fryer to 350°Fahrenheit. In a bowl, mix the coconut oil, seasonings, and butter.

2.   Coat the pork chops with this mixture.

3.   Place the chops on the grill pan of your air fryer and cook them for 8-minutes per side.

NUTRITION: Calories: 356, Total Fat: 30g, Carbs: 2.3g, Protein: 19g

132. Honey Ginger Salmon Steaks

Cooking Time: 10 minutes Servings: 2

INGREDIENTS

- 2salmon steaks
- 2tablespoons fresh ginger, minced
- 2garlic cloves, minced
- ¼ cup honey
- 1/3 cup orange juice
- 1/3 cup soy sauce
- 1lemon, sliced

DIRECTIONS

1.   Mix all the ingredients in a bowl. Marinate the salmon in the sauce for 2-hours in the fridge.

2.   Add the marinated salmon to air fryer at

395°Fahrenheit for 10-minutes.

3.   Garnish with fresh ginger and lemon slices.

NUTRITION: Calories: 514, Total Fat: 22g, Carbs: 39.5g, Protein: 41g

133. Rosemary & Lemon Salmon

Cooking Time: 10 minutes Servings: 2

INGREDIENTS

- 2salmon fillets
- Dash of pepper
- Fresh rosemary, chopped
- 2slices of lemon

DIRECTIONS:

1. Rub the rosemary over your salmon fillets, then season them with salt and pepper, and place lemon slices on top of fillets.

2. Place in the fridge for 2-hours. Preheat your air fryer to 320°Fahrenheit.

3. Cook for 10-minutes.

NUTRITION: Calories: 363, Total Fat: 22g, Carbs: 8g, Protein: 40g

134. Fish with Capers & Herb Sauce

Cooking Time: 15 minutes Servings: 4

INGREDIENTS

- 2cod fillets
- ¼ cup almond flour
- 1teaspoon Dijon Mustard
- 1egg
- Sauce:
- 2tablespoons of light sour cream
- 2teaspoons capers
- 1tablespoon tarragon, chopped
- 1tablespoon fresh dill, chopped
- 2tablespoons red onion, chopped
- 2tablespoons dill pickle, chopped

DIRECTIONS

1. Add all of the sauce ingredients into a small mixing bowl and mix until well blended then place in the fridge.

2. In a bowl mix Dijon mustard and egg and sprinkle the flour over a plate.

3.   Dip the cod fillets first into the egg and coat, then dip them into the flour, coating them on both sides.

4.   Preheat your air fryer to 300° Fahrenheit, place fillets into air fryer and cook for 10- minutes.

5.   Place fillets on serving dishes and drizzle with sauce and serve.

NUTRITION: Calories: 198, Total Fat: 9.4g, Carbs: 17.6g, Protein: 11g

135. Lemon Halibut Cooking Time: 20 minutes Servings: 4

INGREDIENTS

- 4halibut fillets
- 1egg, beaten
- 1lemon, sliced
- Salt and pepper to taste
- 1tablespoon parsley, chopped

DIRECTIONS

1.   Sprinkle the lemon juice over the halibut fillets. In a food processor mix the lemon slices, salt, pepper, and parsley.

2.   Take fillets and coat them with this mixture; then dip fillets into beaten egg.

3.   Cook fillets in your air fryer at

350° Fahrenheit for 15-minutes.

NUTRITION: Calories: 48,   Total Fat: 1g, Carbs: 2.5g, Protein: 9g

136. Fried Cod & Spring Onion Cooking Time: 20 minutes Servings: 4

INGREDIENTS

- 7-ounce cod fillet, washed and dried
- Spring onion, white and green parts, chopped
- A dash of sesame oil
- 5tablespoons light soy sauce
- 1teaspoon dark soy sauce
- 3tablespoons olive oil
- 5slices of ginger
- 1cup of water
- Salt and pepper to taste

DIRECTIONS

1. Season the cod fillet with a dash of sesame oil, salt, and pepper. Preheat your air fryer to 356°Fahrenheit. Cook the cod fillet in air fryer for 12- minutes. For the seasoning sauce, boil water in a pan on the stovetop, along with both light and dark soy sauce and stir. In another small saucepan, heat the oil and add the ginger and white part of the spring onion. Fry until the ginger browns, then remove the ginger and onions. Top the cod fillet with shredded

green onion. Pour the oil over the fillet and add the seasoning sauce on top.

NUTRITION: Calories: 233, Total Fat: 16g, Carbs: 15.5g, Protein: 6.7g

SEAFOOD
RECIPES

352. Garlic Shrimp Bacon Bake Preparation time: 10 minutes Cooking time: 8 minutes

Servings: 4

INGREDIENTS

- ¼ cup butter
- 2Tbsp minced garlic
- 1pound shrimp, peeled and cleaned
- ¼ tsp ground black pepper
- ½ cup cooked, chopped bacon
- 1/3 cup heavy cream
- ¼ cup parmesan cheese

DIRECTIONS:

1. Preheat your air fryer to 400 degrees F and grease an 8x8 inch baking pan.

2. Add the butter and shrimp to the pan and place in the air fryer for 3 minutes. Remove the pan from the air fryer.

3. Add the remaining ingredients to the pan and return to the air fryer to cook for another 5 minutes.

The mix should be bubbling and the shrimp should be pink.

4.   Serve with zucchini noodles or enjoy plain.

NUTRITION: Calories 350, Total Fat 27g, Saturated Fat 15g, Total Carbs 3g, Net Carbs 3g, Protein 36g, Sugar 0g, Fiber 0g, Sodium 924mg, Potassium 16g

353.   Gruyere Shrimp Bacon Bake

Preparation time: 10 minutes Cooking time: 10 minutes Servings: 4

INGREDIENTS

*   ¼ cup butter

*   2Tbsp minced garlic

*   1pound shrimp, peeled and cleaned

*   ¼ tsp ground black pepper

*   ½ cup cooked, chopped bacon

*   1/3 cup heavy cream

*   ¼ cup parmesan cheese

- ½ cup gruyere cheese, grated

DIRECTIONS:

1.   Preheat your air fryer to 400 degrees F and grease an 8x8 inch baking pan.

2.   Add the butter and shrimp to the pan and place in the air fryer for 3 minutes. Remove the pan from the air fryer.

3.   Add the remaining ingredients to the pan and return to the air fryer to cook for another 5 minutes. The mix should be bubbling and the shrimp should be pink.

4.   Sprinkle the gruyere over the shrimp and return to the air fryer for another 2 minutes to brown the top of the cheese.

5.   Serve with zucchini noodles or enjoy plain.

NUTRITION: Calories 410, Total Fat 32g, Saturated Fat 18g, Total Carbs 4g, Net Carbs 3g, Protein 38g, Sugar 0g, Fiber 0g, Sodium 988mg, Potassium 24g

354. Cajun Shrimp Bacon Bake Preparation time: 10 minutes Cooking time: 10 minutes

Servings: 4

INGREDIENTS

- ¼ cup butter
- 2Tbsp minced garlic
- 1pound shrimp, peeled and cleaned
- ½ tsp Cajun seasoning
- ½ cup cooked, chopped bacon
- 1/3 cup heavy cream
- ¼ cup parmesan cheese

DIRECTIONS:

1.   Preheat your air fryer to 400 degrees F and grease an 8x8 inch baking pan.

2.   Add the butter and shrimp to the pan and place in the air fryer for 3 minutes. Remove the pan from the air fryer.

3.   Add the remaining ingredients to the pan and return to the air fryer to cook for another 5 minutes. The mix should be bubbling and the shrimp should be pink.

4.   Serve with zucchini noodles or enjoy plain.

NUTRITION: Calories 352, Total Fat 27g, Saturated Fat 15g, Total Carbs 3g, Net Carbs 3g, Protein 36g, Sugar 0g, Fiber 0g, Sodium 930mg, Potassium 18g

355. Garlic Shrimp Prosciutto Bake

Preparation time: 10 minutes Cooking time: 10 minutes Servings: 4

INGREDIENTS

- ¼ cup butter
- 2Tbsp minced garlic
- 1pound shrimp, peeled and cleaned
- ¼ tsp ground black pepper
- 2oz thinly sliced, shredded prosciutto
- 1/3 cup heavy cream
- ¼ cup parmesan cheese

DIRECTIONS:

1.   Preheat your air fryer to 400 degrees F and grease an 8x8 inch baking pan.

2.   Add the butter and shrimp to the pan and place in the air fryer for 3 minutes. Remove the pan from the air fryer.

3.   Add the remaining ingredients to the pan and return to the air fryer to cook for another 5 minutes. The mix should be bubbling and the shrimp should be pink.

4.   Serve with zucchini noodles or enjoy plain.

NUTRITION: Calories 358, Total Fat 27g, Saturated Fat 15g, Total Carbs 3g, Net Carbs 3g, Protein 36g, Sugar 0g, Fiber 0g, Sodium 1026mg, Potassium 16g

356. Garlic Shrimp Tuna Bake Preparation time: 10 minutes Cooking time: 10 minutes Servings: 4

INGREDIENTS

- ¼ cup butter
- 2Tbsp minced garlic
- 1pound shrimp, peeled and cleaned
- ¼ tsp ground black pepper
- 1tin canned tuna, drained well
- 1/3 cup heavy cream
- ¼ cup parmesan cheese

DIRECTIONS:

1.   Preheat your air fryer to 400 degrees F and grease an 8x8 inch baking pan.

2.   Add the butter and shrimp to the pan and place in the air fryer for 3 minutes. Remove the pan from the air fryer.

3.   Add the remaining ingredients to the pan and return to the air fryer to cook for another 5 minutes. The mix should be bubbling and the shrimp should be pink.

4.   Serve with zucchini noodles or enjoy plain.

NUTRITION: Calories 376, Total Fat 30g, Saturated Fat 15g, Total Carbs 3g, Net Carbs 3g, Protein 43g, Sugar 0g, Fiber 0g, Sodium 924mg, Potassium 16g

357. Jalapeno Tuna Melt Cups

Cooking time: 20 minutes Servings: 7

INGREDIENTS

- 5oz canned tuna, drained
- 2eggs
- ¼ cup sour cream
- ¼ cup mayonnaise
- ¾ cup shredded cheddar cheese
- ¾ cup pepper jack cheese
- ¼ tsp salt
- ¼ tsp ground black pepper
- 1Tbsp parsley, chopped
- ½ cup jalapeno slices

DIRECTIONS:

1.   Preheat your air fryer to 325 degrees F and grease a muffin tin or individual muffin cups-whichever option fits in your air fryer better.

2.   In a large bowl, combine the tuna, mayonnaise, sour cream, both kinds of grated cheese, parsley, jalapeno slices, salt, and pepper.

3.   Scoop the mix into the prepared muffin tin, filling each cup to the top.

4.   Bake in the air fryer for 20 minutes or until the tops are golden brown.

5.   Place on a slice of keto bread, serve with keto crackers or enjoy plain with a spoon!

NUTRITION: Calories 167, Total Fat 13g, Saturated Fat 3, Total Carbs 2g, Net Carbs 1g, Protein 9g, Sugar 2g, Fiber 0g, Sodium 321mg, Potassium 197g

358. Herbed Tuna Melt Cups Preparation time: 10 minutes Cooking time: 20 minutes Servings: 7

Preparation time: 10 minutes

INGREDIENTS

•   5oz canned tuna, drained

•   2eggs

•   ¼ cup sour cream

- ¼ cup mayonnaise

- ¾ cup shredded cheddar cheese

- ¾ cup pepper jack cheese

- ¼ tsp salt

- ¼ tsp ground black pepper

- 1Tbsp parsley, chopped

- 1tsp fresh chopped rosemary

- 1tsp fresh chopped basil

DIRECTIONS:

1.	Preheat your air fryer to 325 degrees F and grease a muffin tin or individual muffin cups- whichever option fits in your air fryer better.

2.	In a large bowl, combine the tuna, mayonnaise, sour cream, both kinds of grated cheese, parsley, rosemary, basil, salt, and pepper.

3.	Scoop the mix into the prepared muffin tin, filling each cup to the top.

4.	Bake in the air fryer for 20 minutes or until the tops are golden brown.

5.	Place on a slice of keto bread, serve with keto crackers or enjoy plain with a spoon!

NUTRITION: Calories 163, Total Fat 13g, Saturated Fat 3, Total Carbs 1g, Net Carbs 1g, Protein 9g, Sugar 1g, Fiber 0g, Sodium 325mg, Potassium 197g

359. Cajun Tuna Melt Cups Preparation time: 10 minutes Cooking time: 20 minutes Servings: 7

INGREDIENTS

- 5oz canned tuna, drained

- 2eggs
- ¼ cup sour cream
- ¼ cup mayonnaise
- ¾ cup shredded cheddar cheese
- ¾ cup pepper jack cheese
- ¼ tsp salt
- ½ tsp Cajun seasoning
- 1Tbsp parsley, chopped

DIRECTIONS:

1.   Preheat your air fryer to 325 degrees F and grease a muffin tin or individual muffin cups-whichever option fits in your air fryer better.

2.   In a large bowl, combine the tuna, mayonnaise, sour cream, both kinds of grated cheese, parsley, Cajun seasoning, salt, and pepper.

3.   Scoop the mix into the prepared muffin tin, filling each cup to the top.

4.   Bake in the air fryer for 20 minutes or until the tops are golden brown.

5.   Place on a slice of keto bread, serve with keto crackers or enjoy plain with a spoon!

NUTRITION: Calories 161, Total Fat 13g, Saturated Fat 3, Total Carbs 1g, Net Carbs 1g, Protein 9g, Sugar 1g, Fiber 0g, Sodium 321mg, Potassium 197g

360. Cheddar Tuna Melt Cups Preparation time: 10 minutes Cooking time: 20 minutes Servings: 7

INGREDIENTS

- 5oz canned tuna, drained
- 2eggs
- ¼ cup sour cream
- ¼ cup mayonnaise
- 1½ cups shredded cheddar cheese
- ¼ tsp salt

- ¼ tsp ground black pepper
- 1Tbsp parsley, chopped

DIRECTIONS

1.   Preheat your air fryer to 325 degrees F and grease a muffin tin or individual muffin cups-whichever option fits in your air fryer better.

2.   In a large bowl, combine the tuna, mayonnaise, sour cream, cheese, parsley, salt and pepper.

3.   Scoop the mix into the prepared muffin tin, filling each cup to the top.

4. Bake in the air fryer for 20 minutes or until the tops are golden brown.

5. Place on a slice of keto bread, serve with keto crackers or enjoy plain with a spoon!

NUTRITION: Calories 160, Total Fat 13g, Saturated Fat 3, Total Carbs 1g, Net Carbs 1g, Protein 9g, Sugar 1g, Fiber 0g, Sodium 321mg, Potassium 197g

348. Salmon Fish Sticks Preparation time: 10 minutes Cooking time: 10 minutes Servings: 4

INGREDIENTS

- 1pound salmon filets
- ¼ cup mayonnaise
- 2Tbsp mustard
- ½ tsp salt
- ½ tsp ground black pepper
- 1½ cups ground pork rinds
- 2Tbsp whole milk

DIRECTIONS:

1.   Preheat your air fryer to 400 degrees F and line your air fryer tray with foil and spray with cooking grease.

2.   Dry the salmon filets by patting with a paper towel. Cut the fish into strips about 1 inch wide and two inches long.

3.   In a small bowl, combine the mustard, mayo and milk and stir together well.

4.   In a separate bowl, combine the ground pork rinds, salt and pepper.

5.   Dip the fish strips into the mayonnaise mix and then into the pork rind mix, coating the fish completely. Place it on the prepared tray when done and repeat with the remaining fish sticks.

6.   Place the tray in the air fryer and bake the fish for 5 minutes, flip and bake for another 5
        minutes Servings while hot!

NUTRITION: Calories 282, Total Fat 18g, Saturated Fat 5g, Total Carbs 1g, Net Carbs 0g, Protein 27g, Sugar 0g, Fiber 1g, Sodium 664mg, Potassium 68g

349. Cajun Salmon Fish Sticks Preparation time: 10 minutes Cooking time: 10 minutes Servings: 4

INGREDIENTS

- 1pound salmon

- ¼ cup mayonnaise

- 2Tbsp mustard

- ½ tsp salt

- 1tsp Cajun seasoning

- 1½ cups ground pork rinds

- 2Tbsp whole milk

DIRECTIONS:

1.   Preheat your air fryer to 400 degrees F and line your air fryer tray with foil and spray with cooking grease.

2.   Dry the salmon filets by patting with a paper towel. Cut the fish into strips about 1 inch wide and two inches long.

3.   In a small bowl, combine the mustard, mayo and milk and stir together well.

4.   In a separate bowl, combine the ground pork rinds, Cajun seasoning, and salt.

5. Dip the fish strips into the mayonnaise mix and then into the pork rind mix, coating the fish completely. Place it on the prepared tray when done and repeat with the remaining fish sticks.

6. Place the tray in the air fryer and bake the fish for 5 minutes, flip and bake for

another 5 minutes Servings while hot!

NUTRITION: Calories 288, Total Fat 18g, Saturated Fat 5g, Total Carbs 1g, Net Carbs 0g, Protein 27g, Sugar 0g, Fiber 1g, Sodium 676mg, Potassium 68g

350. Bacon Wrapped Fish Sticks Preparation time: 10 minutes Cooking time: 18 minutes

Servings: 4

INGREDIENTS

- 1pound cod

- ¼ cup mayonnaise

- 2Tbsp mustard

- ½ tsp salt

- ½ tsp ground black pepper

- 1½ cups ground pork rinds

- 2Tbsp whole milk

- ½ pound bacon, uncooked, strips

DIRECTIONS:

1. Preheat your air fryer to 400 degrees F and line your air fryer tray with foil and spray with cooking grease.

2. Dry the cod filets by patting with a paper towel. Cut the fish into strips about 1 inch wide and two inches long.

3. In a small bowl, combine the mustard, mayo and milk and stir together well.

4. In a separate bowl, combine the ground pork rinds, salt and pepper.

5. Dip the fish strips into the mayonnaise mix and then into the pork rind mix, coating the fish completely. Place it on the prepared tray when done and repeat with the remaining fish sticks.

6. Wrap each fish stick in the bacon and place back onto the tray.

7. Place the tray in the air fryer and bake the fish for 10 minutes, flip and bake for

another 8 minutes or until the bacon is brown and crispy. Serve while hot!

NUTRITION: Calories 310, Total Fat 24g, Saturated Fat 5g, Total Carbs 1g, Net Carbs 0g, Protein 34g, Sugar 0g, Fiber 1g, Sodium 899mg, Potassium 112g

351. Keto Tuna Melt Cups Preparation time: 10 minutes Cooking time: 20 minutes Servings: 7

INGREDIENTS

- 5oz canned tuna, drained
- 2eggs
- ¼ cup sour cream
- ¼ cup mayonnaise
- ¾ cup shredded cheddar cheese
- ¾ cup pepper jack cheese
- ¼ tsp salt
- ¼ tsp ground black pepper
- 1Tbsp parsley, chopped

DIRECTIONS:

1. Preheat your air fryer to 325 degrees F and grease a muffin tin or individual muffin cups-whichever option fits in your air fryer better.

2. In a large bowl, combine the tuna, mayonnaise, sour cream, both kinds of grated cheese, parsley, salt and pepper.

3. Scoop the mix into the prepared muffin tin, filling each cup to the top.

4. Bake in the air fryer for 20 minutes or until the tops are golden brown.

5. Place on a slice of keto bread, serve with keto crackers or enjoy plain with a spoon!

NUTRITION: Calories 160, Total Fat 13g, Saturated Fat 3, Total Carbs 1g, Net Carbs 1g, Protein 9g, Sugar 1g, Fiber 0g, Sodium 321mg, Potassium 197g

Poultry Recipes

423. Herbed Turkey Preparation time: 10 minutes
Cooking time: 30 minutes Servings: 6

INGREDIENTS

- 1pound turkey breast, skinless, boneless and sliced
- 1tablespoon basil, chopped
- 1tablespoon coriander, chopped
- 1tablespoon oregano, chopped
- 1tablespoon olive oil
- ½ cup chicken stock
- Juice of 1 lime
- Salt and black pepper to the taste

DIRECTIONS

1. In the air fryer's pan, mix the turkey with the basil and the other ingredients and cook at 370 degrees F for 30 minutes.

2. Divide the mix between plates and serve.

NUTRITION: Calories 281, Fat 7, Fiber 8, Carbs 20, Protein 28

424. Chicken Wings and Sprouts Preparation time: 10 minutes Cooking time: 25 minutes

Servings: 4

INGREDIENTS

• 2pounds chicken wings, halved

• 1cup Brussels sprouts, trimmed and halved

• 1cup tomato sauce

• 1teaspoon hot sauce

• Salt and black pepper to the taste

• 1teaspoon coriander, ground

• 1teaspoon cumin, ground

• 1tablespoon cilantro, chopped

DIRECTIONS

1. In the air fryer's pan, mix the chicken with the sprouts and the other ingredients, toss, cook at 380 degrees F for 25 minutes, divide between plates and serve.

NUTRITION: Calories 271, Fat 7, Fiber 6, Carbs 14, Protein 20

425. Thyme Turkey Preparation time: 10 minutes Cooking time: 30 minutes Servings: 4

INGREDIENTS

• 2pounds turkey breast, skinless, boneless and cubed

• 2tablespoons thyme, chopped

• Juice of 1 lime

• 1teaspoon olive oil

• Salt and black pepper to the taste

• 2tablespoons tomato paste

• ½ cup chicken stock

- 1tablespoon chives, chopped

DIRECTIONS

1. In the air fryer's pan, mix the turkey with the thyme and the other ingredients, introduce the pan in the air fryer and cook at 380 degrees F for 30 minutes.

2. Divide the mix between plates and serve.

NUTRITION: Calories 271, Fat 11, Fiber 7, Carbs 17, Protein 20

426. Cumin Chicken Preparation time: 10 minutes Cooking time: 30 minutes Servings: 4

INGREDIENTS

- 1tablespoon olive oil
- 1pound chicken breast, skinless, boneless and cubed
- Salt and black pepper to the taste
- 1teaspoon cumin, ground
- 3spring onions, chopped

- ½ cup tomato sauce
- 1cup chicken stock
- ½ tablespoon chives, chopped

DIRECTIONS:

1.   In the air fryer's pan, mix the chicken with the oil and the other ingredients and toss.

2.   Introduce the pan in the air fryer and cook at 380 degrees F for 30 minutes.

3.   Divide everything between plates and serve.

NUTRITION: Calories 261, Fat 11, Fiber 6, Carbs 19, Protein 17

427. Ground Chicken and Chilies Preparation time: 10 minutes Cooking time: 30 minutes

Servings: 4

INGREDIENTS

• 2pounds chicken breast, skinless, boneless and ground

• 1yellow onion, minced

• 1teaspoon chili powder

• 1teaspoon sweet paprika

• Salt and black pepper to the taste

• 1tablespoon olive oil

• 4ounces canned green chilies, chopped

• A handful parsley, chopped

DIRECTIONS

1. In the air fryer's pan, mix the chicken with the onion, chili powder and the other ingredients, introduce the pan in the air

fryer and cook at 370 degrees F for 30 minutes.

2.   Divide into bowls and serve.

428. Chopped Chicken Olive Tomato Sauce

Preparation time: 10 minutes Cooking time: 30 minutes Servings: 4

INGREDIENTS

* 500 g chicken cutlet
* 2minced shallots+1 degermed garlic clove
* 75 g of tomato sauce + 15 g of 30% liquid cream
* 1bay leaf+salt+pepper+1 tsp Provence herbs
* 20pitted green and black olives

DIRECTION:

1.   Cut the chicken cutlets into strips and put them in the fryer basket with the garlic and the shallots. Do not put oil. Salt/pepper.

2.   Set the timer and the temperature to 10- 12 minutes at 200°C

3.   Add the tomato sauce, the cream, the olives, the bay leaf, and the Provence herbs. Salt if necessary. Mix with a wooden spoon.

4.   Close the air fryer and program 20 minutes at 180°C.

5.   Eat hot with rice or pasta.

NUTRITION: Calories 220.2 Fat 7.0 g Carbohydrate 8.5 g Sugars 4.5 g Protein28.9 g Cholesterol 114.8 mg

429. Chicken Thighs in Coconut Sauce, Nuts

Preparation time: 10 minutes Cooking time: 30 minutes

Servings: 4

INGREDIENTS

•   8skinless chicken thighs

•   2chopped onions

•   25ml of coconut cream + 100 ml of coconut milk

- 4tbsp coconut powder + 1 handful of dried fruit mix+ 5 dried apricots, diced + a few cashew nuts and almonds

- Fine salt + pepper

DIRECTION:

1. Put the onions, chopped with the chicken thighs, in the air fryer (without oil). Add salt and pepper. Program 10 minutes at 200°C.

2. Stir alone with a wooden spoon.

3. Add coconut cream and milk, coconut powder, dried fruits, and apricots. Get out if necessary. Continue cooking by programming 20 minutes at 200°C. You don't have anything to do; it cooks alone, without any problem.

4. With the tongs, remove the bowl and serve hot with rice, vegetables, Chinese noodles.............. A delight. Perfect kitchen

NUTRITION: Calories 320.4 Fat 11.6 g Carbohydrate 9.0 g Sugars 2.1 g Protein44.0 g Cholesterol 102.7 mg

430. Forest Guinea Hen Preparation time: about 15 minutes Cooking time: 1 h 15 - 1 h 30 Servings: 4

INGREDIENTS

•   A beautiful guinea fowl farm weighing 1 to 1.5 kilos

•   100g of dried or fresh porcini mushrooms according to the season

•   8large potatoes Béa

•   1plate

•   2cloves of garlic

•   1shallot

•   Chopped parsley

•   A pinch of butter

•   Vegetable oil

•   Salt and pepper

DIRECTION:

1.   Put the dried mushrooms in water to rehydrate them or simply clean them if they are fresh porcini mushrooms. Peel the potatoes and cut them finely. Chop the garlic and parsley and set aside.

2.   Prepare the guinea fowl by cutting the neck and removing all the giblets inside. Garnish with stuffed dough, garlic cloves and parsley.

3.   Place guinea fowls in the air fryer at 2000C without oil of sufficient capacity. Simply add the butter knob and a tablespoon of cooking oil. Allow approximately one hour of cooking per kilo, so you will have to check after a certain period.

4.   When the guinea fowl is ready, prepare the porcini mushrooms in the oil-free fryer by adding the shallot. This preparation is very fast, and you should not forget salt and pepper.

5.   When everything is ready, place each of the preparations in the air fryer, sprinkle with the cooking juices and cook for another 15 minutes.

6.   Serve hot to enjoy all the flavors of the dish.

NUTRITION: Calories 110 Fat 2.5g Carbohydrate 0g Sugars 0g Protein 21g Cholesterol 63mg

431. Fried and Crispy Chicken

Preparation time: 15 minutesCooking time: 35-40 minutes Servings: 4

INGREDIENTS

- 4chicken breasts
- 1tbsp olive oil
- 1tbsp breadcrumbs
- 1tbsp of a spice mixture
- Salt
- 250g of potatoes per person

DIRECTION:

2.   Cut chicken breasts into 4 slices

3.   Mix them with the other ingredients so that the chicken is perfectly covered with the preparation.

4.   Peel and cut the potatoes in the same way as the fries, trying to make a regular cut to cook better.

5.   Place the strips in the air fryer without oil and cook at 200oC for 15 to 20 minutes to get a crispy chicken.

6.   For French fries, wait 30 minutes to cook.

NUTRITION: Calories 227 Carbohydrates 23g Fat 18g Sugars 0g Protein 12g Cholesterol 63mg

432. Orange Turkey Bites Preparation time: 10-20 Cooking time: 15-30

Servings: 8

INGREDIENTS

- 750 g turkey
- 1shallot
- 2oranges
- Thyme to taste
- 1tsp oil
- Salt and pepper to taste

DIRECTION:

2. Cut the turkey into pieces and peel the oranges, cutting the skin into strips.

3. Put the chopped shallot, the orange peel, the thyme, and the oil in the basket of the preheated air fryer at 150 for 5 minutes. Brown all for 4 min.

4. Add ½ glass of water, lightly floured turkey, salt, and pepper; simmer for 6 more minutes.

5.   Then add the orange juice and cook at 2000C for 15 minutes until a thick juice is obtained.

6.   Serve garnished with some thyme leaves and slices of orange.

NUTRITION: Calories 80 Fat 5g Carbohydrates 1g Sugar 0g Protein 7g Cholesterol 25mg

433. Chicken Thighs with Potatoes Preparation time: 0-10 Cooking time: 45-60

Servings: 6

INGREDIENTS

- 1kg chicken thighs
- 800g of potatoes in pieces
- Salt to taste
- Pepper to taste
- Rosemary at ease
- 1clove garlic

DIRECTION:

2.   Preheat the air fryer at 1800C for 15 minutes.

3.   Place the chicken thighs in the basket and add the previously peeled and washed potatoes, add a clove of garlic, rosemary sprigs, salt, and pepper.

4.   Set the temperature 2000C and cook everything for 50 min. Mix 3-4 times during cooking (when they are well browned on the surfaceand chicken 1-2 times.

NUTRITION: Calories 419.4 Fat 9.5 g Carbohydrate 44.8 g Sugars2.0 g Protein39.1 g Cholesterol 115.8 mg

434. Chicken Blanquette With Soy

Preparation time: 10-20

Cooking time: 15-30 Servings:

INGREDIENTS

- 600g Chicken breast

- 300g Potatoes

- 100g Bean sprouts

- 150g Broth

- 50g Onion

- 1tsp Olive oil

- 25g Soy sauce

DIRECTION:

1.   Cut the meat and potatoes into pieces.

2.   Pour the sliced oil and onion into the bottom of the tank, close the lid.

3.   Set the air fryer at 1500C to brown for 5 minutes.

4.   Add the floured chicken, potatoes, broth, salt, and pepper and cook for another 13 minutes.

5.   Then pour the sprouts and the soy sauce and cook for another 10 minutes.

NUTRITION: Calories 250 Carbohydrates 19g Fat 11g Sugars 7g Protein 16g Cholesterol 0mg

419. Meatballs and Sauce Preparation time: 10 534. Beef with Sesame and Ginger

Preparation time: 10 minutes Cooking time: 23 minutes Servings: 4-6

INGREDIENTS

- ½ cup tamari or soy sauce
- 3tbsp olive oil
- 2tbsp toasted sesame oil
- 1tbsp brown sugar
- 1tbsp ground fresh ginger
- 3cloves garlic, minced

- 1to 1½ pounds skirt steak, boneless sirloin, or low loin

DIRECTION:

1. Put together the tamari sauce, oils, brown sugar, ginger, and garlic in small bowl. Add beef to a quarter-size plastic bag and pour the marinade into the bag. Press on the bag as much air as possible and seal it.

2.   Refrigerate for 1 to 1½ hours, turning half the time. Remove the meat from the marinade and discard the marinade. Dry the meat with paper towels. Cook at a temperature of 350°F for 20 to 23 minutes, turning halfway through cooking.

NUTRITION: Calories: 381 Fat: 5g Carbohydrates: 9.6g Protein: 38g Sugar: 1.8g Cholesterol: 0mg

535. Katsu Pork Preparation time: 10 minutes Cooking time: 14 minutes Servings: 2

INGREDIENTS

• 170g pork chops, boneless

• 56g of breadcrumbs

• 3g garlic powder

• 2g onion powder

• 6g of salt

• 1g white pepper

• 60g all-purpose flour

• 2eggs, shakes

• Nonstick Spray Oil

DIRECTION:

1.   Place the pork chops in an airtight bag or cover them with a plastic wrap.

2.   Crush the pork with a meat roller or hammer until it is 13 mm thick.

3.   Combine the crumbs and seasonings in a bowl. Leave aside.

4.   Pass each pork chop through the flour, then soak them in the beaten eggs and finally pass them through the crumb mixture.

5.   Preheat the air fryer set the temperature to 180°C.

6.   Spray pork chops on each side with cooking oil and place them in the preheated air fryer.

7.   Cook the pork chops at 180°C for 4 minutes.

8.   Remove them from the air fryer when finished and let them sit for 5 minutes.

9.   Cut them into pieces and serve them.

NUTRITION: Calories: 820   Fat: 24.75g
Carbohydrates: 117g Protein: 33.75g Sugar: 0g
Cholesterol: 120mg

536. Pork on A Blanket Preparation time: 5 minutes Cooking time: 10 minutes Servings: 4

INGREDIENTS

- ½ puff pastry sheet, defrosted
- 16thick smoked sausages
- 15ml of milk

DIRECTION:

1.   Preheat la air fryer to 200°C and set the timer to 5 minutes.

2.   Cut the puff pastry into 64 x 38 mm strips.

3.   Place a cocktail sausage at the end of the puff pastry and roll around the sausage, sealing the dough with some water.

4.   Brush the top (with the seam facing downof the sausages wrapped in milk and place them in the preheated air fryer.

5.   Cook at 200°C for 10 minutes or until golden brown.

NUTRITION: Calories: 242 Fat: 14g Carbohydrates: 0g Protein: 27g Sugar: 0g Cholesterol: 80mg

Vegetables
Recipes

1. Salsa Zucchini

Preparation time: 5 minutes

Cooking time: 20 minutes Servings: 4

INGREDIENTS

- 1POund zucchinis, roughly sliced
- 1Cup mild salsa
- 1Red onion, chopped
- Salt and black pepper to the taste
- 2tablespoons lime juice
- 2tablespoons olive oil
- 1TEAspoon coriander, ground

DIRECTIONS

1. In a pan that fits your air fryer, mix the zucchinis with the salsa and the other ingredients, toss, introduce in the fryer and cook at 390 degrees F for 20 minutes.

2. Divide the mix between plates and serve. NUTRITION: Calories 150, Fat 4, Fiber 2, Carbs 4, Protein 5

2.Green Beans and Olives

Preparation time: 5 minutes Cooking time: 20 minutes Servings: 4

INGREDIENTS

- 1POund green beans, trimmed and halved
- 1Cup black olives, pitted and halved
- 1Cup kalamata olives, pitted and halved
- 1Red onion, sliced
- 2tablespoons balsamic vinegar
- 1TAblespoon olive oil
- 3garlic cloves, minced
- ½ cup tomato sauce

DIRECTIONS

1. In a pan that fits your air fryer, mix the green beans with the olives and the other ingredients, toss, put the pan in the fryer and cook at 350 degrees F for 20 minutes.

2. Divide the mix between plates and serve. NUTRITION: Calories 180, Fat 4, Fiber 3, Carbs 5, Protein 6

3. Spicy Avocado Mix

Preparation   time: 5   minutes
      Cookingtime: 15 minutes Servings: 4

INGREDIENTS:

- 2small avocados, pitted, peeled and cut into wedges
- 1TAblespoon olive oil
- Zest of 1 lime, grated
- Juice of 1 lime
- 1TAblespoon avocado oil
- A pinch of salt and black pepper
- ½ teaspoon sweet paprika

DIRECTIONS

1.   In a pan that fits the air fryer, mix the avocado with the lime juice and the other ingredients, put the pan in your air fryer and cook at 350 degrees F for 15 minutes.

2.   Divide the mix between plates and serve.
NUTRITION: Calories 153, Fat 3, Fiber 3, Carbs 4, Protein 6

4.Spicy Black Beans

Preparation time: 5 minutes Cooking time: 20 minutes Servings: 4

INGREDIENTS

- 2cups canned black beans, drained
- 1TAblespoon olive oil
- 1TEAspoon chili powder
- 2red chilies, minced
- Apinch of salt and black pepper
- ¼ cup tomato sauce

DIRECTIONS

1.   In a pan that fits the air fryer, mix the beans with the oil and the other ingredients, toss, put the pan in the air fryer and cook at 380 degrees F for 20 minutes.

2.   Divide between plates and serve.

NUTRITION: Calories 160, Fat 4, Fiber 3, Carbs 5,

Protein 4

5.Cajun Tomatoes and Peppers

Preparation time: 4 minutes Cooking time: 20 minutes Servings: 4

INGREDIENTS

- 1TAblespoon avocado oil
- ½ pound mixed bell peppers, sliced
- 1POund cherry tomatoes, halved
- 1Red onion, chopped
- A pinch of salt and black pepper
- 1TEAspoon sweet paprika
- ½ tablespoon Cajun seasoning

DIRECTIONS

1.   In a pan that fits the air fryer, combine the peppers with the tomatoes and the other ingredients, put the pan it in your air fryer and cook at 390 degrees F for 20 minutes.

2.   Divide the mix between plates and serve. NUTRITION: Calories 151, Fat 3, Fiber 2, Carbs 4, Protein 5

6.Olives and Sweet Potatoes

Preparation   time: 5   minutes   Cooking time: 25 minutes Servings: 4

INGREDIENTS

- 1POund sweet potatoes, peeled and cut into wedges

- 1Cup kalamata olives, pitted and halved

- 1TAblespoon olive oil

- 2tablespoons balsamic vinegar

- A bunch of cilantro, chopped

- Salt and black pepper to the taste

- 1TAblespoon basil, chopped

DIRECTIONS

1. In a pan that fits the air fryer, combine the potatoes with the olives and the other ingredients and toss.

2. Put the pan in the air fryer and cook at 370 degrees F for 25 minutes.

3. Divide between plates and serve. NUTRITION: Calories 132, Fat 4, Fiber 2, Carbs 4, Protein 4

7.Spinach and Sprouts

Preparation time: 5 minutes Cooking time: 20 minutes Servings: 4

INGREDIENTS

- 1POund Brussels sprouts, trimmed and halved
- ½ pound baby spinach
- 1TAblespoon olive oil
- Juice of 1 lime
- Salt and black pepper to the taste
- 1TAblespoon parsley, chopped DIRECTIONS:

1. In the air fryer's pan, mix the sprouts with the spinach and the other ingredients, toss, put the pan in the air fryer and cook at 380 degrees F for 20 minutes.

2. Transfer to bowls and serve.

NUTRITION: Calories 140, Fat 3, Fiber 2, Carbs 5, Protein 6

Dessert and snacks

1.Banana Cake

Preparation time: 10 minutes Cooking time: 1-hour Servings: 4

INGREDIENTS

- 1Cup water, for the pressure cooker
- 1ANd ½ cups sugar
- 2cups flour
- 4bananas, peeled and mashed
- 1TEAspoon cinnamon powder
- 1TEAspoon nutmeg powder

DIRECTIONS

1.   In a bowl, mix sugar with flour, bananas, cinnamon and nutmeg, stir, pour into a greased cake pan and cover with tin foil.

2.   Add the water to your pressure cooker, add steamer basket, add cake pan, cover and cook on High for 1 hour.

3.   Slice, divide between plates and serve cold. NUTRITION: Calories 300, Fat 10, Fiber 4, Carbs 45, Protein

2.Pineapple Pudding

Preparation time: 10 minutes Cooking time: 5 minutes Servings: 8

INGREDIENTS

- 1TAblespoon avocado oil
- 1Cup rice
- 14ounces milk
- Sugar to the taste
- 8ounces canned pineapple, chopped

DIRECTIONS

1. In your pressure cooker, mix oil, milk and rice, stir, cover and cook on High for 3 minutes.

2. Add sugar and pineapple, stir, cover and cook on High for 2 minutes more.

3. Divide into dessert bowls and serve.

NUTRITION: Calories 154, Fat 4, Fiber 1, Carbs

14, Protein

3.Blueberry Jam

Preparation time: 10 minutes Cooking time: 11 minutes Servings: 2

INGREDIENTS

- ½ pound blueberries
- 1/3 pound sugar
- Zest from ½ lemon, grated
- ½ tablespoon butter
- A pinch of cinnamon powder

DIRECTIONS

1. Put the blueberries in your blender, pulse them well, strain, transfer to your pressure cooker, add sugar, lemon zest and cinnamon, stir, cover and simmer on sauté mode for 3 minutes.

2. Add butter, stir, cover the cooker and cook on High for 8 minutes.

3. Transfer to a jar and serve.

NUTRITION: Calories 211, Fat 3, Fiber 3, Carbs 6, Protein

4.   Bread Pudding

Preparation time: 10 minutes

Cooking   time: 20   minutes   Servings: 4
INGREDIENTS:

- 2egg yolks
- 1ANd ½ cups brioche cubed
- 1Cup half and half
- ¼ teaspoon vanilla extract
- ½ cup sugar
- 1TAblespoon butter, soft
- ½ cup cranberries
- 2cups water
- 3tablespoons raisins
- Zest from 1 lime, grated

DIRECTIONS

1.   In a bowl mix, egg yolks with half and half, cubed brioche, vanilla extract, sugar, cranberries, raisins and lime zest, stir, pour into a baking dish greased with the butter and leave aside for 10 minutes.

2.   Add the water to your pressure cooker, add the steamer basket, add the dish, cover and cook on High for 20 minutes.

3.   Serve this cold.

NUTRITION: Calories 162, Fat 6, Fiber 7, Carbs 9, Protein

5.Coconut Cream and Cinnamon Pudding

Preparation time: 10 minutes Cooking time: 10 minutes Servings: 6

INGREDIENTS

- 2cups coconut cream

- 1TEAspoon cinnamon powder

- 6tablespoons flour

- 5tablespoons sugar

- Zest of 1 lemon, grated

- 2cups water, for the pressure cooker

DIRECTIONS

1.   Set your pressure cooker on sauté mode, add coconut cream, cinnamon and orange zest, stir, simmer for a couple of minutes, transfer to a bowl and leave aside.

2.   Add flour and sugar, stir well and divide this into ramekins.

3.   Add the water to your pressure cooker, add steamer basket, add ramekins, cover pot, cook on Low for 10 minutes and serve cold.

NUTRITION: Calories 170, Fat 5, Fiber 2, Carbs 8, Protein 10

5.Plum Jam

Preparation time: 20 minutes Cooking time: 8 minutes Servings: 12

INGREDIENTS

- 3pounds plums, stones removed and roughly chopped
- 2tablespoons lemon juice
- 2pounds sugar
- 1TEAspoon vanilla extract
- 3ounces water

DIRECTIONS

1. In your pressure cooker, mix plums with sugar and vanilla extract, stir and leave aside for 20 minutes

2. Add lemon juice and water, stir, cover and cook on High for 8 minutes.

3. Divide into bowls and serve cold.

NUTRITION: Calories 191, Fat 3, Fiber 4, Carb 12,

Protein 17

6.Cranberry Bread Pudding

Preparation time: 10 minutes Cooking time: 15 minutes Servings: 2

INGREDIENTS

- 2egg yolks
- 1ANd ½ cups bread, cubed
- 1Cup heavy cream
- Zest from ½ orange, grated
- Juice from ½ orange
- 2teaspoons vanilla extract
- ½ cup sugar
- 2cups water
- 1TAblespoon butter
- ½ cup cranberries

DIRECTIONS

1.   In a bowl, mix egg yolks with bread, heavy cream, orange zest and juice, vanilla extract, sugar, butter and cranberries, stir and pour into a baking dish.

2.   Add the water to your pressure cooker, add the steamer basket, add baking dish, cover cooker and cook on High for 15 minutes.

3.   Divide between 2 plates and serve cold.

NUTRITION: Calories 189, Fat 3, Fiber 1, Carbs 4, Protein 6

CPSIA information can be obtained
at www.ICGtesting.com
Printed in the USA
LVHW051914120121
676284LV00005B/574